Distribution, publication, and copying in any form are prohibited and subject to damages.

TEN HYPNOSES

Copying, publishing, and sharing with third parties are only permitted with the written consent of the author. Please observe the notes on copyright and usage.

Distribution, publication, and copying in any form are prohibited and subject to damages.

Copying, publishing, and sharing with third parties are only permitted with the written consent of the author. Please observe the notes on copyright and usage.

Distribution, publication, and copying in any form are prohibited and subject to damages.

Ingo Michael Simon

TEN HYPNOSES

14

Panic Attacks

Copying, publishing, and sharing with third parties are only permitted with the written consent of the author. Please observe the notes on copyright and usage.

Distribution, publication, and copying in any form are prohibited and subject to damages.

© 2024 Ingo Michael Simon
All rights reserved.
Independently published
www.ingosimon.com

Important Notes for Urgent Attention:
The contents of this book are based on the practical experiences of the author with hypnosis applications and psychotherapy in a trance state. Although the author has strived for the utmost care, errors or misunderstandings in the presentation cannot be completely excluded. Therapeutic work with people and the application of hypnosis are solely the responsibility of the hypnotist. It cannot be ruled out that parts of this book may be misunderstood or that the application of a presented procedure may cause an undesirable reaction in the client. The author also assumes no co-responsibility if work with a client is carried out with reference to the statements in this book.

The Author:
Ingo Michael Simon studied psychology and education and is a hypnotherapist with practices in southwestern Germany and Switzerland. With the help of hypnosis-supported psychotherapy, he primarily treats people with persistent psychological conditions. His practice focuses on anxiety disorders, pathological compulsions, and psychosomatic illnesses. His therapeutic offerings mainly include classical and modern hypnosis applications and the dreamland therapy he developed himself.

Copying, publishing, and sharing with third parties are only permitted with the written consent of the author. Please observe the notes on copyright and usage.

Distribution, publication, and copying in any form are prohibited and subject to damages.

Notes on Copyright and Usage

Copying, publishing, and sharing with third parties is prohibited and only permitted with the written consent of the author. Please observe the following copyright and usage guidelines.

This work has been carefully crafted and created to the best of the author's knowledge and personal experience. It comprises text templates and application guidelines for professional hypnosis sessions. The author is a licensed psychotherapist with extensive experience in psychotherapy, coaching, and personal training using hypnotic techniques and methods. Nevertheless, the author and the publisher assume no liability for the accuracy of information, instructions, and advice, nor for any typographical errors. The author and publisher accept no responsibility or liability for the application of these texts and recommendations with clients or patients, nor for any potential consequences or unexpected reactions. It is expressly noted that the application of therapeutic and advisory techniques and formulations lies solely and entirely within the responsibility of the practitioner. This also applies to adherence to the boundaries of legally regulated medical and therapeutic practices. The fact that a book containing action proposals is freely available for sale does not imply that its application with clients or patients is permitted for everyone.

Distribution, publication, and copying in any form are prohibited and subject to damages.

Copying, publishing, and sharing with third parties are only permitted with the written consent of the author. Please observe the notes on copyright and usage.

Distribution, publication, and copying in any form are prohibited and subject to damages.

Table of Contents

Introduction 9

#1 11

#2 16

#3 21

#4 27

#5 32

#6 37

#7 42

#8 47

#9 52

#10 57

Overview of All Titles in the Series "Ten Hypnoses" 62

Copying, publishing, and sharing with third parties are only permitted with the written consent of the author. Please observe the notes on copyright and usage.

Distribution, publication, and copying in any form are prohibited and subject to damages.

Copying, publishing, and sharing with third parties are only permitted with the written consent of the author. Please observe the notes on copyright and usage.

Introduction

The series "Ten Hypnoses" is very well known in Germany, Austria, and Switzerland as a collection of texts for therapeutic work and is used by numerous psychotherapeutic practices, doctors, therapists, coaches, and other helping professionals. I am pleased to now be able to offer these texts in other countries as well.

Most therapists have their own methods for inducing and deepening trance as well as for exiting trance. Therefore, I have focused on the main part of the hypnosis. The texts in this book can be integrated as the main part into any hypnosis process.

The texts in this collection use various hypnosis techniques. I will not explain these in detail, as I assume that users have the appropriate training. It is also not necessary to understand the exact structure or functioning of the different parts. The texts can simply be read aloud, and they will have their effect.

Decide for yourself which text best suits your client or patient at any given time. You can also combine passages from different texts. It is not about using all ten hypnoses in sequence. It is a selection of possibilities.

I want to emphasize that books cannot replace therapy. Psychotherapy or other therapeutic treatments involve much more. A careful diagnosis is the necessary basis for deciding on the use of methods, including whether hypnosis or one of my texts should be used. Even in this case, preparatory discussions, follow-up discussions during the session, and of course, a therapeutic concept for the sequence of sessions and the content approaches are essential parts of therapy. This cannot and should not be achieved with a collection of texts.

In any case, I wish you much success in your work and I am pleased if my text templates can contribute in a small way.

Ingo Michael Simon

#1

You have decided to gain control over your fear ... ... This is best achieved when you manage to perceive other feelings that are also present more clearly ... ... Within you, there is also a feeling of strength, of your own power ... ... Power and strength within you ... ... The strength to shape your life ... ... The strength to decide for yourself what should and can be ... ... Strength that helps you be stronger than the fear ... ... You know the anticipation of fear, which over time has grown so great that it became worse than the actual panic attack, which occurred much less frequently than the anticipation of fear ... ... So today you will reorganize ... ... Today, you will change your thoughts ... ... You have the feeling of strength within you, so from today on you will use it more intensely ... ...

... ... You formulate the thought that with your own power and strength you can stand up to emerging fear ... ... As soon as it is possible to feel your own strength even in the face of emerging fear, you will get through the difficult situations ... ... So you let this thought of your own strength become clear ... ... like a big headline in your head ... ... I am strong and conquer the fear ... ... like a headline you read and are immediately excited by ... ... It is written within you ... ... I am strong and conquer the fear ... ... This sentence becomes a very decisive one because it becomes your creed ... ... I am strong and conquer the fear ... ... Every thought begins with this one creed ... ... I am strong and conquer the fear ... ... When your thoughts align with this, your mind ... ... then your entire organism can align with it, your body and your feeling ... ... and your mind has long decided that it should be so ... ... It is your will, you want to control the fear ... ... You want to master the fear ... ... You want to conquer the fear ... ... You make yourself big in front of your fear, big and strong ... ... because this makes your fear smaller and smaller ... ... You are bigger than the fear ... ... You are also stronger than the fear ... ... This thought becomes the first and most important thought of the day ... ... I am strong and conquer the fear ... ... And from your thoughts, this message now flows into your body ... ... Your mind informs your body about the intense idea of your strength ... ... Your mind informs your body about the new truth of your own strength and power ... ... Your body takes in this message and finds the strength in every part of your body ... ... every single cell ... ... and there too, your strength grows ... ... Your body feels the new strength within you ... ... the strength that can and will conquer every fear ... ... Maybe you already feel the change in your body, this new strength ... ... maybe you will feel it a bit later because right now it's all about relaxation ... ... But your body feels this strength and lets it grow stronger and stronger ... ... So your thoughts have already adjusted to strength and power to master the fear ... ... and now your body has also adjusted to strength and power to master the fear ... ... Now you are ready for the third important step, the change in feelings ... ... If you now focus entirely on your actual feeling, you will feel relaxation and calm ... ... There is no fear now, only relaxation and calm ... ... and within this calm lies the strength ... ... in this very calm lies a deep strength within you ... ... Strength within you ... ... Your body informs your emotions that strength and power are becoming noticeable ... ... Every cell in your body helps to make this new strength and power very clear in your feeling ... ... You can feel your strength if you focus entirely on your body ... ... The more you succeed in consciously feeling your body now, the more the clear feeling of strength within you will arise ... ... You may already notice and perceive it now ... ... now or in a few moments ... ... Strength within you ... ...

... ... So your mind continues to send the thought ... ... I am strong and conquer the fear ... ... Your thoughts increasingly align with this new truth ... ... I am strong and conquer the fear ... ... Your body takes in this message and makes a tangible truth in every cell out of it ... ... Your body also says ... ... I am strong and conquer the fear ... ... Your body ingrains this thought into every single cell ... ... I am strong and conquer the fear ... ... And also deep within your emotions, deep within you, this thought appears as a new and intense feeling ... ... I am strong and conquer the fear ... ... You have this feeling within you ... ... I am strong and conquer the fear ... ... It becomes a clearer and stronger feeling that you can clearly perceive ... ... I am strong and conquer the fear ... ...

... ... That's good ... ... Take your time to let everything take effect ... ... Mind, body, and feelings realign and help you conquer the fear ... ... Everything aligns so that you can actually feel this strength ... ... as a feeling, as an emotion

... ... Everything aligns so that your body has this power and can call upon it ... ... can make it available to you anytime ... ... Everything aligns so that you can always think this thought of your own strength with great conviction and confidence ... ... that you can always feel this thought of your own power and might like an inner echo ... ... I am strong and conquer the fear ... ... I am strong and conquer the fear ... ... I am strong and conquer the fear ... ...

You can amplify the effect even more by saying this decisive sentence out loud ... ... In the morning when you wake up, you start with it ... ... You get up and say ... ... I am strong and conquer the fear ... ... When you look in the mirror in the morning, say it again ... ... I am strong and conquer the fear ... ... and whenever you say this sentence, you immediately feel the new strength within you, because your thoughts, your body, and your feeling align with it and make it a reality ... ... I am strong and conquer the fear ... ... Whenever you want to become even stronger, you say your new creed out loud ... ... I am strong and conquer the fear ... ... and immediately you can feel your own strength ... ... Strength that can conquer the fear ... ... Strength that can conquer the fear … … just like here and today … … exactly like here and today … …

#2

You have decided to do something about your fear ... ... You have always wanted to fight it, have already tried many things, have gone to doctors and therapists ... ... You have now decided to do something with the help of hypnosis ... ... Today, we will focus on the fear of expectation ... ... You know this fear, this constant fear that a panic attack could break out ... ... This expectation has often been worse than the actual panic because the expectation has constantly accompanied you ... ... Now it is time to end this ... ... You want to experience your everyday life with ease again ... ... You want to be free again ... ... free in your thoughts ... ... free in your ideas ... ... free in your feelings ... ... that is what matters ... ...

... ... You resolve to gradually let go of the expectation of fear and at the same time gradually replace it with the expectation of lightness ... ... Maybe you think it won't be so easy, but maybe it is easier than you thought ... ... Focus on your breathing and imagine that you can exhale the expectation of fear and at the same time inhale the feeling of lightness ... ... This is more than an imagination ... ... Let's start ... ... Breathe slowly and evenly ... ... deeply in and slowly and long out ... ... good ... ... When exhaling, you let go of the expectation of fear ... ... You let go of the expectation ... ... and when inhaling, you take in the idea of lightness with the breath ... ... Maybe you have already noticed that you actually feel a bit lighter when inhaling ... ... Pay attention to your body feeling when inhaling ... ... Your upper body moves upwards, expands, and indeed feels a bit lighter ... ... and now you can let go of the expectation of fear and take in lightness ... ...

... ... [Speak in the rhythm of the client's breathing; when exhaling, say "Expectation" and when inhaling "Lightness." For the client, in addition to the idea of exhaling the expectation of fear, the associative connection "Expectation-Lightness" is formed, which should replace the previous association "Expectation-Fear."] ... ...

... ... Let go of the expectation ... ... Inhale lightness ... ... Let go of the expectation ... ... Inhale lightness ... ... [Client exhales] ... Expectation ... ... [Client inhales] ... Lightness ... ... [Client exhales] ... Expectation ... ... [Client inhales] ... Lightness ... ... [Client exhales] ... Expectation ... ...

[Client inhales] ... Lightness ... ... [Client exhales] ... Expectation ... ... [Client inhales] ... Lightness ... ... So easy it can be ... ... Your subconscious stores this rhythm ... ... So you can just let your thoughts drift and trust that deep inside everything is being reorganized ... ... completely by itself, because your subconscious now knows what to do ... ... with every breath ... ... [Client exhales] ... Expectation ... ... [Client inhales] ... Lightness ... ... without thinking, everything continues ...

... ... You are adjusting internally ... ... your subconscious gradually lets go of the expectation of fear ... ... with each breath a bit more ... ... and at the same time, the feeling of lightness spreads within you ... ... You can feel the relief if you focus on your body ... ... You feel the relaxation and with each breath in the lightness of your body ... ...

... ... [Client exhales] ... Expectation ... ... [Client inhales] ... Lightness ... ... [Client exhales] ... Expectation ... ... [Client inhales] ... Lightness ... ... good ... ... Your body has already stored it and knows that the expectation of fear is let go with every exhale ... ... and with every inhale, the idea of lightness is taken in ... ... with every inhale, the feeling of lightness becomes clearer ... ...

...... With this exercise, you inform your entire body about a simple principle that it continues for you, especially when you no longer think about it ...... even in sleep, when you are in deep rest, your body keeps letting go of the expectation of fear ...... and keeps setting up the feeling of relief and lightness ...... this feeling that makes fear impossible because you feel the inner lightness deeply ...... with every breath ......

...... Let go of the expectation ...... Inhale lightness ...... Let go of the expectation ...... Inhale lightness ...... [Client exhales] ... Expectation ...... [Client inhales] ... Lightness ... . [Client exhales] ... Expectation ...... [Client inhales] ... Lightness ...... [Client exhales] ... Expectation ...... [Client inhales] ... Lightness ...... [Client exhales] ... Expectation ...... [Client inhales] ... Lightness ...... So easy it can be ...... Your subconscious stores this rhythm ...... So you can just let your thoughts drift and trust that deep inside everything is being reorganized ...... completely by itself, because your subconscious now knows what to do .... with every breath ...... [Client exhales] ... Expectation ... ... [Client inhales] ... Lightness ...... without thinking, everything continues ...

And tonight, while you sleep, your subconscious does exactly the same for you ... ... breathes away the fear for you and builds up relief ... ... inner lightness for you ... ... the deeper you sleep, the easier it is for your subconscious to really build lightness ... ... inner lightness ... ... and fear fades away ...

#3

The following variant of a hypnosis main part works with an anchor in the form of sunglasses with colored lenses. An anchor is a trigger that is supposed to create a specific feeling or evoke a specific thought. We want to help the client maintain an anxiety-free state and counteract the onset of a panic attack with the help of sunglasses. Glasses in the colors yellow, orange, or blue are best suited. In a state of relaxation, no fear can be felt, so we use a deep state of relaxation to set up the glasses as an anchor. We let the client open their eyes and look through the colored lenses in trance. Suggestively, we connect this color perception with the feeling of relaxation that is currently prevailing. In everyday life, the client should then wear the glasses continuously for a few weeks when going out of the house. The color perception should help to prevent the fear from arising. This approach may sound strange. Just try out the colored glasses. You might be surprised at how well they are accepted and how well they usually work. However, they are not suitable for emergency intervention. If the fear is *already present, they do not unfold the necessary effect. But don't worry. Your anxiety patients will gladly wear the sunglasses. By the way, you don't need special (and usually very expensive) color therapy glasses. Any sports glasses for joggers or cyclists are suitable. They are already available from 5 euros. Simply give your client the task of getting such glasses and bringing them along. They should wear them throughout the session.*

You have firmly resolved to master the fear ... ... You know the sudden fear that has paralyzed you so often ... ... You can train to control emerging fear, but you can do more ... ... You can ensure that it doesn't even come up in the first place ... ... You can avert it before it really arises ... ... For this, it is helpful to reach a very deep state of relaxation now ... ... You allow yourself to relax even more now ... ... to sink even deeper ... ... deeper and deeper ... ... into a wonderful state of calm ... ... of deep inner calm ... ... and if you are tired, then imagine you are starting to dream ... ... as if you were about to fall asleep ... ... just fall asleep ... ... to dream a beautiful dream ... ... in wonderful images that can feel really good to you ... ... beautiful images of calm and relaxation ... ... beautiful images of peace and stillness ... ... Everything becomes calm within you ... ... everything becomes very calm ... ... That's right ... ... that's good ... ... just calm and relaxation ... ... deep calm and deep relaxation ... ... Now you feel good ... ... now nothing can burden or disturb you ... ... and if there should still be any disturbing thought, you simply breathe it out ... ... It is then as if you could breathe out any tension and any thought that could still be in the way and thereby let go ... ... with every breath until you really feel free and relaxed ... ... So breathe out for your inner calm ... ... Breathe out for your inner peace ... ... Breathe out for your relaxation ... ... Breathe out the fear ... ... Breathe out any thought of fear ... ... Breathe out any memory of fear ... ... Breathe out and find calm ... ... Find deeper and deeper calm and relaxation ... ... deeper and deeper calm and relaxation ... ... So beautifully relaxed, everything is fine ... ... Your body can now learn to maintain this state, relaxed and free from fear, permanently ... ... Your entire organism can learn this, right now ... ... Focus on your feeling ... ... on this feeling of calm and relaxation that you are feeling right now ... ... The more you focus on the feeling of calm, the clearer it becomes ... ... and now prepare to open your eyes and perceive the color of calm and serenity ... ... I will count to three, then you open your eyes ... ...

... ... [Count with a calm voice, no pressure and no raised tone; it's not about ending the trance, but about fractionation.] ... ... one ... ... two ... ... three ... ... Open your eyes and perceive the color of calm and serenity ... ... Perceive this beautiful sun yellow (yellow/orange/blue) very clearly and let this beautiful color flow deep into your consciousness ... ... It becomes the color of your calm and serenity ... ... good ... ... very good ... ... Now close your eyes again and feel the beautiful sun yellow (yellow/orange/blue) deep within you ... ... good ... ... very good ... ...

Now feel the inner calm ... ... You can still feel it, maybe even more clearly than before ... ... and at the same time, your deep inner self learns that this beautiful color is the color of your serenity ... ... the color of your inner calm ... ... This learning happens all by itself ... ... deep within you, it has already happened, your organism already knows that with the perception of the color sun yellow (yellow/orange/blue) the feeling of calm and serenity is so important that you must feel it clearly ... ... So your own body immediately sends you this feeling of calm and serenity as soon as you perceive the color sun yellow ... ... Let your body once again absorb this beautiful effect and make it real ... ...

I will count once more to three for you, then you can open your eyes again and absorb the beautiful color of your calm and serenity even more ... ... [Count with a calm voice, no pressure and no raised tone; it's not about ending the trance, but about fractionation.] ... ... one ... ... two ... ... three ... ... Open your eyes and perceive the color of calm and serenity ... ... Perceive this beautiful sun yellow (yellow/orange/blue) very clearly and let this beautiful color flow deep into your consciousness ... ... It becomes the color of your calm and serenity ... ... good ... ... very good ... ... Now close your eyes again and feel the beautiful sun yellow (yellow/orange/blue) deep within you ... ... good ... ... very good ... ...

Your body now knows that there is your color of calm, which is also your anti-fear color ... ... and whenever you wear the glasses you are now looking through, and then perceive this beautiful color, your organism immediately remembers the important calm and serenity you need ... ... and whenever you look through the glasses, your deep inner self immediately provides you with the feeling of calm and serenity, as well and as strongly as it can ... ... With all its strength, calm arises within you when looking through the glasses you are now wearing ... ... Every day calm and serenity ... ... every day ... ... just like now ... ... exactly like now ... ...

#4

The following variant of a hypnosis main part works with an anchor in the form of a key. An anchor is a trigger that is supposed to create a specific feeling or evoke a specific thought. We want to help the client maintain an anxiety-free state and counteract the onset of a panic attack with the help of a key. I always use a slightly antique-looking cabinet key for this. They are available in any well-stocked hardware store for 1-2 euros. In a state of relaxation, no fear can be felt, so we use a deep state of relaxation to set up the key as an anchor. Relaxation and fear cannot exist simultaneously. Trance and fear can! So it is important that a state of real relaxation is present. Symbolically, we let the client lock the fear in a chest, which remains with the therapist. The client should carry the key for this locked and thus controlled fear. Especially at the beginning, it is useful for them to carry the key in their hand when leaving the house to also be connected to the anchor in their consciousness. This alleviates the fear of expectation more quickly. However, the key is also not suitable as an *emergency intervention. If the fear is already present, it does not unfold the necessary effect. Behavioral therapy techniques help more for acute self-control of fear than hypnosis. It is also good if you have a small chest to which the key fits so that the chest with the locked fear actually remains with the therapist. But it also works as a visualization.*

You have been dealing with the fear for some time now ... ... You can already grasp it much better, maybe even understand it to some extent ... ... Often we cannot really understand our fears but only observe how they behave or change ... ... Repressing fear has not really worked, because it has always found its way out ... ... You know that you will let go of the fear deep within you over time ... ... that it will dissolve as you better understand yourself and work on what has frightened you in your life ... ... The panic attacks come suddenly, but there were also other fears in your life ... ... Fears you had to deal with, some of which you were able to overcome ... ... some you couldn't really work on and just held out until it became calmer again ... ... So something always remains within us unresolved and sometimes it breaks through ... ... But first, it is important to be able to control the fear, to be able to steer it somehow ... ... and then, in a next step, you can dare to dissolve the old fears and concerns ... ... and thereby dissolve the fear step by step ... ... but today we want to control the fear first ... ... as if you could lock it up and only let it out when you want to ... ... controlled fear ... ... For this, you now find even deeper relaxation because in relaxation the fear cannot harm you ... ... you cannot even feel it in relaxation ... ... You now feel relaxation ... ... You have taken the time to come to rest step by step, so you can also come to even more rest ... ... so you can also find even more inner relaxation ... ... find more calm ... ... find more peace ... ... You feel the relaxation of your body ... ... and if you think your body should relax even deeper, then let it happen ... ... Focus simply on the spot in your body or the area that should relax more ... ... Direct your attention there and think the word calm ... ... once again ... ... calm ... ... good ... ... calm ... ... Your body follows your thoughts and wishes and sets this calm there ... ... try it again ... ... Choose a spot in your body or a part of your body that should relax deeper ... ... direct your attention there and think calm ... ... once again ... ...

calm ... ... good ... ... calm ... ... Now let go of all thoughts, just let them drift ... ... now it's only about your calm ... ... because now in calm you can control the fear ... ... You can imagine the fear flowing into a small chest ... ...

... [If you have a small chest to which the key fits, place it opened next to the client, preferably before the hypnosis session. But it works just as well as a visualization that the client visualizes.] ...

The fear flows into the opened chest that is right next to you ... ... Imagine you are breathing out the fear ... ... It flows out of you with the exhale as the wind of fear and flows into the small opened chest ... ... You can stand next to yourself in your mind's eye and watch the fear flow into the chest ... ... with every breath ... ... until it is completely in there ... ... In a few moments, this has already happened ... ... Your fear is in the small chest, which I now close for you ... ...

... [Close the chest audibly and give the key to the client in the next sequence. Without a real chest, they can hold the key in their hand from the beginning.] ...

... ... The fear is now in the chest ... ... I now give you the key to the chest / You feel the key in your hand ... ... You thereby have control over the fear because it cannot leave the chest as long as you hold the key ... ... Only you can now decide when the fear can be there to look at and work with it ... ... You have locked it up ... ... You hold the key to the fear in your hand ... ... The fear can no longer decide for itself ... ... The key in your hand keeps the fear in the chest, far away from you ... ... At this moment, you are free from any fear ... ... You feel good, you are well ... ... You have the key in your hand and are free from fear ... ...

... ... The key in your hand always reminds you that you have control over the fear ... ... As long as you hold the key in your hand, you are free from fear and stay free from fear ... ... So you can simply take the key with you and carry it in your hand when you leave your home ... ... As soon as you feel the key in your hand, you also feel your strength and courage because fear is under control ... ... Fear is under your control ... ... every day just like now ... ... exactly like now ... ... You hold the key firmly in your hand ...

#5

You are here today to work on your fear ... ... You have already tried some things to make it smaller or to get rid of it ... ... In the process, you have made some progress, maybe you have learned to handle the fear quite well ... ... But you want to work on it further, make it even smaller ... ... ideally, make it disappear completely ... ... to be completely free again ... ... completely free from fear ... ... and also free from the fear of fear, because you know that well too ... ... Often it was that you anxiously waited for when the next panic attack would come ... ... Then it was not even the actual panic attack that was the main problem, but the waiting for it ... ... that was also a fear that led to constant fear ... ... But you have decided to change that ... ... to fight against it with all your strength and conviction and to replace fear with a new feeling ... ... with the feeling of lightness ... ... Maybe you are also wondering how quickly it can go to really free yourself from fear ... ... maybe you are thinking about how quickly it might go to leave the fear behind ... ... to live completely without fear, with a good feeling ... ... with the feeling of lightness that automatically arises when fear steps aside ... ... and while you are still thinking about how quickly it might go to be free from fear, your subconscious concentrates more and more on this idea of fear, on the memory of fear ... ... Now, in this state of relaxation and calm, you cannot develop fear and that is good ... ... now there can also be no fear of fear and that is very good ... ... because now you can calmly think about the fear ... ... because now you can look at it calmly ... ... and that is how it can always be ... ... stay calm at the thought of fear ... ... Over time, it has come that the fear hangs like a big headline over your everyday life, like a headline ... ... You can also imagine this headline now, maybe like on a huge, white screen, on which in big letters the word fear is written ... ... Deep within you, it is so that a part of you has always stared at this screen since the time of the panic attacks and has made the word fear grow larger and larger ... ... But today you are allowed to stare at this screen and you will feel no fear because that is not possible in relaxation ... ... So look and imagine the word fear very clearly, as if it were written on a large, white screen ... ... Fear ... ... While doing so, you realize that the fear of the next fear, the anticipatory fear, has become so strong because there was no other way but to constantly think about the fear ... ... or about the possible fear that didn't always really come through ... ... While you were busy with so many things in everyday life and had to do so much, the fear could grow larger and larger ... ... could make the word on your inner screen so big and thick ... ... It can also go the other way around ... ... what can gain great significance internally can also become smaller again ... ... because now you have time to deal only with this term ... ... Fear ... ... Now you are not distracted by everyday life, now you are in a state of inner calm, in a state of beautiful trance ... ... so now you can make the term fear smaller ... ... Maybe you have already noticed that I have said the word fear many times ... ... yet you are feeling calm and relaxed now, you can just think about fear, without problems ... ... So it is possible to constantly talk about fear and always think about fear without feeling fear ... ... It is possible and you can feel it at this moment ... ... Thus, the inner fear has already become more neutral ... ... But there is more ... ... Look at the word fear and let it become smaller ... ... Let it shrink slowly before your inner eye ... ... The clearer you imagine the word fear, the smaller it becomes before your inner eye and thus smaller in your feeling ... ... In front of your eyes, the fear on the inner screen becomes smaller and smaller ... ... always smaller ... ... as if the word were moving further and further into the distance ... ... The individual letters become smaller when you look directly at the word ... ... look directly at the fear ... ... It is as if you are hypnotizing the fear with your gaze and making it slowly disappear ... ... The letters collapse, shrink and shrink ... ... The clearer and more intense you look at the screen, the smaller the fear, which was written there, becomes ... ... always smaller and smaller ... ... until it is only tiny and thin letters that you can hardly recognize ... ... So your screen becomes brighter and eventually really white again ... ... This way, soon new letters and words can appear on it ... ... maybe the word freedom, which slowly grows larger ... ... It stands in the same place where the fear once stood, which is disappearing more and more ... ... So the term freedom spreads out ... ... and with it the feeling of freedom ... ... Freedom within you ...

Your subconscious ingrains this ... ... So you can make fear disappear more and more intensely by simply imagining the screen and making the term fear smaller ... ... Then you simply replace it with the word freedom ... ... You simply take a piece of paper every day and write in big letters freedom on it and immediately your subconscious remembers to make the possible fear very small and to let the feeling of freedom become very strong ... ...

#6

Fear is not unchangeable ... ... You can influence it when you let inner images emerge in a state of calm, images that will then accompany you naturally and effortlessly in everyday life ... ... You have images of fear that have often accompanied you ... ... But from now on, they will be images of security ... ... Images that can help you prevent fear from arising and also let go of emerging fear ... ... before it can become truly threatening ... ... You can imagine fear as a fragile glass ball that you have been carrying around in a backpack ... ... and sometimes this ball has broken in your backpack, allowing the fear to escape ... ... The same mental image of a backpack that you carry with you can now help you carry security and thus have the feeling of security ready to access ... ... So imagine you are packing your backpack of security ... ... First, you pack padding for the glass ball of fear ... ... something that can protect the glass ball so it no longer breaks ... ... Think about what that could be, perhaps some foam or cotton to wrap the ball of fear well ... ... Then think about what symbol or object best represents protection for you ... ... maybe a lucky charm or an amulet ... ... a special gemstone ... ... Choose a symbol that means protection and put it in your backpack ... ... This object will additionally protect the ball of fear, ensuring the fear stays securely in the ball ... ... But you can achieve even more ... ... You can use the feeling of your own power ... ... your power over fear ... ... your own strength and might ... ... the power that can help you control and manage emerging fear or even the anticipation of fear ... ... Choose a symbol or an object that best represents your power ... ... maybe a card with the words "I am strong" ... ... or a scepter that signifies power and authority ... ... maybe a crown that makes you a king or queen and thus symbolizes your own power ... ... Choose an object of power and put it in the backpack ... ... Pack this symbol of your own power so you can feel it when things get difficult ... ... so you can counter a possible emerging fear with your own strength ... ... Thus, you have already taken care of protection and your power ... ... Just as you imagine packing something into your backpack, symbols for the feelings you need most to overcome fear, deep inside you, the change that helps you is happening ... ... because all the images we imagine become feelings and convictions deep inside us ... ... In the past, the anticipation of fear became a reality, the expectation of the next fear attack ... ... But today it is different ... ... Today, security becomes reality ... ... Today, protection becomes reality ... ... and thus you can control fear ... ... But you can do even more ... ... Protection and security are important ... ... Your power is important ... ... But the feeling of lightness is also important, because in the feeling of lightness, fear cannot even arise ... ... So you also pack lightness into your backpack and carry inner lightness with you all the time ... ... Choose a symbol or object that best represents lightness ... ... Decide on a symbol of lightness ... ... perhaps a feather that is so light it can float in the wind and not fall to the ground ... ... perhaps a small balloon that is so light it can fly away in the wind ... ... It could carry away any emerging fear and make you feel free ... ... Maybe you have a completely different symbol or object of lightness ... ... a symbol that best represents lightness for you, whatever it may be ... ... Simply take your best symbol of lightness and pack it in your backpack ... ... Now you already have protection in your backpack ... ... now you already have security in your backpack ... ... Now you already have power in your backpack … … and you have lightness in your backpack … … and the more you pack into your backpack, the more good feelings and aids, the lighter the backpack becomes … … It becomes easier to carry because everything you have put into it helps you let go of fear … … or control and manage it if it arises … … Fear once made your backpack heavy … … but you are making it light now … … You only need the inner vision … … only the images within you … … In a state of relaxation, in a state of pleasant and helpful trance, in which you are currently, the positive and helpful images become reality … … because just as you now have the image of the helpful backpack with the signs and symbols within you, so you have the feelings that you packed into the backpack actually with you in your waking life … … They are available to you to help, because your subconscious knows that you have gathered the helpful feelings and abilities in your inner backpack … … Everything that can free you is within you … … It is only about finding the helpful and strong abilities and feelings when you need them the most … … when fear arises or the anticipation and expectation of fear arises … … With the mental image of the helpful backpack, you can internally sort the helpful images and feelings … … You have bundled them so that they are easier and quicker to access in your waking life and help you out of fear ... ...

This also succeeds in your waking life, especially when you are outside ... ... Then it is as if you are carrying this backpack with freedom in your luggage ... ... If you want, you can take a backpack or a bag with you when you leave your home ... ... Then it is like an outer sign of the packed backpack that helps you control and manage fear ... ... and as soon as even the slightest thought of fear could arise, you remember the packed backpack and know exactly that you have freedom in your luggage ... ... inner and outer freedom ... ... inner and outer freedom ... ...

#7

The following application can be done without an induction into trance and thus works even more effectively. A leg catalepsy (immobility of the extended leg while lying down) is induced, which symbolizes the outer "immobility" or paralysis during a fear attack and the inner immobility of holding onto fear patterns. Reversing the catalepsy symbolizes the release from holding on and thus overcoming fear and paralysis. Symbolically, inner mobility returns with the outer resolution of catalepsy. Of course, the whole process can also be done after an extensive trance induction, but I recommend avoiding that because the catalepsy functioning without (prepared) hypnosis leaves a stronger impression. Experienced hypnotists know: Catalepsy works even without hypnosis, but if it works, it is hypnosis! You probably can't just read the following text like all the others. I still encourage you to try this variant once. It is not about the wording but about the approach. So you don't need to memorize every word.

I want to show you that your feeling of not being able to move during a fear attack or not being able to control the situation is an ingrained belief. A conviction you can let go of to get through your panic attacks and eventually overcome the fear. Your fear has accompanied you for a long time, but it has already become smaller. You have confronted your fear, scrutinized it, and understood a lot, and perhaps some things remain unresolved. Maybe we can't fully understand fear. Maybe everything has its meaning and time. Letting go of fear is easier if you manage to let go of your bad conscience. The bad conscience that arose because you blame yourself for not always having everything under control. Fear often had control over you. You then believed that it couldn't go away easily. But today you want to let it go and with it the bad conscience. You don't need it anymore. You were never to blame for your fear. I now claim that fear is mainly in you because you can't really imagine it can go away or change. You probably can't imagine that you wouldn't be able to move your leg because you suddenly imagine it won't work. You probably don't believe that. You think you can't unlearn something as simple as moving your leg. Alright. I want to show you something that can demonstrate your own thinking. The thinking deep inside you. The unconscious thinking. But you can influence that too. I'll help you with that.

Catalepsy Phase

Now concentrate on your right leg ... ... Now imagine this leg is getting longer and longer. It stretches longer and longer. It gets longer and longer, only in your imagination. The leg becomes two meters long, three meters long. Longer and longer. Imagine it. Your leg becomes five meters long, ten meters long. Always longer. It even becomes a hundred meters long. And it becomes more and more solid. The longer it gets, the more solid your leg becomes. Your leg becomes two hundred meters long. One kilometer. Your leg stretches, becomes longer and longer, ten kilometers long is your leg. It bores through the city. And now imagine that your leg becomes more and more solid the longer it gets, and let it get even longer. Imagine that any attempt to move your leg causes it to become another kilometer longer. And more solid. As soon as you try to lift your leg, it gets even longer and more solid. As soon as you somehow try to lift your leg, it gets even longer and more solid. Try now to lift your leg, and your leg stretches ... Try again. Try to lift your leg, and your leg stretches longer ... Try again, and your leg gets even longer and more solid ... Try again. Your leg remains solid ...

This simple exercise can also be done as a suggestibility test. It works very well and is really achievable without a prior trance induction in a short time. It takes no more than one or two minutes for the leg to stay straight and firm in response to the command to lift it. Simple but effective suggestion!

It doesn't work anymore. You can't do both at the same time. Moving and becoming firmer is not possible. Your belief that your leg is getting longer and firmer keeps it horizontal. If I now tell you that this is not true, that you have just connected two incompatible things, you can simply imagine that your leg will immediately become short and movable the next time you try to move it. Your leg is movable. You just need to know it. Your leg is fully movable. Move your leg.

Now discuss this exercise with your client. Explain to them that their fear paralysis during a panic attack, the inner fear pattern, and the bad conscience are similar. They believe they are unchangeable, immovable like the cataleptic leg, and that they cannot influence them. Repeat the exercise and let the client speak. They should lie down and keep saying: "My leg is getting longer and firmer." Check the catalepsy for them by gently pressing on the leg muscle. Let them keep saying: "When I try to move my leg, it becomes even firmer." They should then try it. It will likely initially lead to catalepsy again, which they can then dissolve themselves by saying: "I can and will now move my leg because it is movable!" Practice a bit with the client until they succeed in inducing and dissolving catalepsy themselves.

Dear readers, try this exercise at least once. It is fun and usually brings an "Aha effect". It shows that belief can work very quickly and clearly, in one direction and then also in the other. Try the exercise on yourself. You will be surprised how well it works in self-suggestion. And how quickly you can also undo the effect. Of course, you can also prevent the effect from the outset. Please try it ...

#8

You want to do something about your fear ... ... There are many types of fear, and most of them are quite normal ... ... when a dangerous situation occurs, we feel fear ... ... Fear can be good to warn us ... ... Then there are fears that slow us down, you know that ... ... You know the sudden fear that becomes intense quickly ... ... But it can also pass just as quickly, you know that too ... ... The time of fear feels endless, but suddenly it gets better, feels lighter ... ... Then you feel that the fear attack is passing ... ... Then your body also changes ... ... In a state of fear, your pulse starts to race, your heart beats faster ... ... everything feels tight, and you can't breathe properly ... ... You know the feeling well because you have experienced it so often ... ... Your body reacts to your feelings, that is normal ... ... and because that is so, you can also change your feelings through the posture and movements of your body ... ... It works both ways ... ... When fear comes, your pulse gets faster, so does your breathing ... ... If you could slow your pulse, the fear would lessen ... ... and that is actually possible ... ... You can slow your breathing and thus also your pulse, which automatically slows down with the breathing ... ... I will show you how it works, and because you are in a state of deep calm, in a state of pleasant trance, it works even better ... ... you free yourself even faster and easier from the fear ... ... Now breathe in slowly while I count to three, then hold your breath briefly and breathe out slowly and long while I count to four ... ... Just follow my voice ... ...

... ... We start ... ... [Make sure the client follows your rhythm. Correct them if necessary.] ... ... Breathe in ... ... one ... ... two ... ... three ... ... Hold ... ... and breathe out ... ... one ... ... two ... ... three ... ... four ... ... and again ... ... Breathe in ... ... one ... ... two ... ... three ... ... Hold ... ... and breathe out ... ... one ... ... two ... ... three ... ... four ... ... and again ... ... [Repeat the process about five to ten times] ... ...

... ... and now imagine the last panic attack exactly ... ... Imagine it and feel the pleasant feeling of calm within you ... ... Breathe in ... ... one ... ... two ... ... three ... ... Hold ... ... and breathe out ... ... one ... ... two ... ... three ... ... four ... ... That's good ... ... You can't feel fear now ... ... Fear and relaxation don't coexist ... ... Now you are relaxed ... ... Fear is impossible ... ... Now you are relaxed ... ... Fear is impossible ... ... Your body is now learning to be without fear ... ... Your entire organism is now learning to be relaxed and free ... ... Breathe in ... ... one ... ... two ... ... three ... ... Hold ... ... and breathe out ... ... one ... ... two ... ... three ... ... four ... ... and again ... ... Breathe in ... ... one ... ... two ... ... three ... ... Hold ... ... and breathe out ... ... one ... ... two ... ... three ... ... four ... ...

... ... The longer your breathing path becomes, the calmer and slower you breathe, the calmer it gets within you ... ... the more and faster the fear fades away ... ... I will continue to count for you, and you will breathe in the rhythm of the numbers ... ... This time I will count to four for inhaling and five steps for exhaling ... ... We start ... ... [Make sure the client follows your rhythm. Correct them if necessary.] ... ... Breathe in ... ... one ... ... two ... ... three ... ... four ... ... Hold ... ... and breathe out ... ... one ... ... two ... ... three ... ... four ... ... five ... ... and again ... ... Breathe in ... ... one ... ... two ... ... three ... ... four ... ... Hold ... ... and breathe out ... ... one ... ... two ... ... three ... ... four ... ... five ... ... and again ... ... [Repeat several times] ... ...

... ... and now imagine the last panic attack exactly ... ... Imagine it and feel the pleasant feeling of calm within you ...

... Breathe in ... ... one ... ... two ... ... three ... ... four ... ... Hold ... ... and breathe out ... ... one ... ... two ... ... three ... ... four ... ... five ... ... That's good ... ... You can't feel fear now ... ... Fear and relaxation don't coexist ... ... Now you are relaxed ... ... Fear is impossible ... ... Now you are relaxed ... ... Fear is impossible ... ... Your body is now learning to be without fear ... ... Your entire organism is now learning to be relaxed and free ... ... Breathe in ... ... one ... ... two ... ... three ... ... four ... ... Hold ... ... and breathe out ... ... one ... ... two ... ... three ... ... four ... ... five ... ... and again ... ... Breathe in ... ... one ... ... two ... ... three ... ... four ... ... Hold ... ... and breathe out ... ... one ... ... two ... ... three ... ... four ... ... five ... ...

Now feel your body ... ... become aware of the deep relaxation that now drives away every thought of fear, makes every thought of fear impossible ... ... Feel the relaxation of your body, which deeply stores this approach ... ... Breathing now makes you free, breathing always makes you free ... ... So now you can control your fear ... ... so well that you no longer feel it ... ... So now you can control your fear every day ... ... so well that you no longer feel it ... ... So now you can even immediately control emerging fear ... ... so well that you no longer feel it ... ...

... ... You feel the change in your body and realize that your body can always show you how you feel in your emotions ... ... especially with emerging feelings of fear ... ... Now you know how to control the emerging fear immediately ... ... You simply breathe in slowly and long, counting to four ... ... and then slowly and long out to five ... ... and fear fades away like now ... ... Fear fades away just like now ... ...

#9

I invite you on a very special journey ... ... a journey that only you can make because only you have access to the world of your own imagination and creativity ... ... to your own dreams ... ... But imagination and reality are very close to each other, so close that we sometimes can't distinguish them ... ... or don't have to distinguish them because every daydream can become reality when the right time comes ... ... Maybe the right time is now, in this very moment ... ... So you focus your attention and mindfulness on the center of your body, where your gut feeling resides, and you imagine sinking into this point with all your awareness ... ... sinking deeper and deeper into yourself to be fully in your feeling ... ... to arrive now in the land of your dreams ... ... The land of your dreams, where anything is possible that you can think of ... ... You arrive in the land of dreams ... ... You stand in the middle of a golden yellow field ... ... a beautiful wheat field that is so vast you can't see the end ... ... You enjoy the warm summer wind on your skin and breathe deeply in and out ... ... and in front of you in the field stand many silver mirrors, large mirrors in which you can see your full reflection ... ... The silver mirrors are lined up side by side, forming a line across the wheat field ... ... You walk very close to look into a mirror ... ... You see your reflection in full size ... ... You recognize your face, your clothes, your hairstyle ... ... And behind you, you can recognize a place or a spot where you had a panic attack that you remember well ... ... It is as if you are looking through a window to see yourself ... ... to observe yourself from the outside, in the land of dreams ... ... Here you are always safe ... ... Here there is no fear or panic ... ... Here there is only you ... ... and you recognize the fear in your reflection ... ... the fear also in your body posture, because you remember how it was during the panic attacks ... ... You were overwhelmed by fear, unable to resist it ... ... But today is different because today you can change something ... ... Today you can go back to the time before the fear ... ... to a time when there might have been fear, but not the overwhelming, uncontrollable fear of panic attacks ... ... And it can be like that again, like back then when there was no panic ... ... Then you walk from mirror to mirror, seeing yourself over and over ... ... Each mirror in the land of dreams represents a month ... ... You want to find the time when everything was still different ... ... maybe you have to go back many months, then it will be many mirrors you walk past and look into ... ... or only a few ... ... With each look into the mirrors you pass by, you realize that you are changing because you are getting younger ... ... even if you only get a few months younger because the panic attacks only got so strong recently, you are changing ... ... maybe your clothes change ... ... your hairstyle ... ... You might become fatter or thinner because you had a different figure back then ... ... and it can also be that you look much younger ... ... You walk past more and more mirrors because your path leads back into the past ... ... if you want, you go very far back into the past ... ... to a time that might be long before the fear, perhaps even many years before ... ... So it may be that you get smaller with time because you go back to your childhood ... ... You keep looking into the mirrors and soon recognize yourself as a child ... ... with that come memories from your childhood ... ... and finally, you just stop and look into the mirror you are standing in front of ... ... You see yourself in the mirror ... ... maybe as an adult or as a teenager ... ... or as a child ... ... You look at yourself ... ... in a time before the panic ... ... But that might not have been a good time ... ... maybe there were other difficulties or challenges ... ... maybe even other fears that you remember now ... ... Then you also see pictures and scenes in the mirror that show you again what was important in your life back then ... ... You go into this mirror yourself to look at that earlier time again ... ... and whether you have arrived in a difficult time or a happy one is not so important ... ... The most important thing is that you have arrived in an earlier time in the land of dreams ... ... your own imagination has brought you here ... ... your deep inner self has brought you to this time ... ... Here you can learn today to be free from fear ... ... Look around and let the images of the earlier time affect you ... ... Where are you? ... ... Who is with you? ... ... What was going on back then? ... ... How did you feel back then? ... ... There are two ways to free yourself from fear today ... ... If you have arrived in a time that was beautiful and light, you can let this good feeling of the past work deeply within you because the land of dreams is the land of feelings, and you can absorb and take your own feeling here ... ... If you have arrived in a difficult time, then realize that the difficult things belong to the past and are no longer important in your present ... ... Then you say goodbye to the past time, which should only remain a memory ... ... So pay attention to your feeling and sense how the time back then feels ... ... Then prepare to either take a good feeling with you or say goodbye to the past time ... ... [Give about half a minute of perceived time, then continue reading] ... ... Now do what is right ... ... take good feelings with you ... ... and say goodbye to the past ... ... and with a big step, you step out of the mirror back onto the golden yellow field ...

Then you lie down in the middle of the field and simply rest ... ... In your mind's eye, you see yourself, free from fear and internally light ... ... In your imagination, you have already let go of the panic ... ... but imagination and reality are very close to each other, and in the land of dreams, both are the same ... ... So you can let go of the fear in your waking life too ... ... You have already let it go there too ... ... Then you think about the fact that the land of dreams is deep within you ... ... It has always been there ... ... I am just telling you about it ...

#10

Sometimes we dream the most impossible things at night ... ... it seems there are no boundaries in dreams, sometimes we can do things that we can't really do in a waking state ... ... or vice versa ... ... It is our feelings that create our imaginations and inner images that can help us learn more about ourselves ... ... understand more about ourselves ... ... be closer to ourselves ... ... It is the same in daydreams ... ... they too have no boundaries ... ... and daydreams also allow us to glimpse deep into our inner selves ... ... into the realm of the unconscious and feelings ... ... And dreams not only reveal a lot about ourselves, but they also create reality ... ... they drive us and change our actions ... ... Thus, dreams can also help us overcome difficult situations ... ... Deep inside, there are a thousand dreams we can dream ... ... a thousand dreams that can help us ... ... Deep inside you, there are a thousand dreams that can help you free yourself from fear ... ... and today, you are experiencing one of those dreams ... ... The wind of your breath brings you to the land of your imagination and creativity ... ... to the land of your dreams ... ...

... ... You stand on sandy ground by the sea ... ... You see the waves running out on the shore and hear the sound of the sea, which sounds like the sound of your breath ... ... The sky is light blue and clear, and you feel the warm wind on your skin ... ... the salty taste of the sea air ... ... Then you see a large rock in the water ... ... far out ... ... You think about the panic ... ... about this overwhelming fear that has often overcome you ... ... You have tried to understand the fear, but it is not always possible to truly understand why and how it originated ... ... You have decided to overcome the fear, to let it go again ... ... You have long searched for the strength you need to do so ... ... and this strength lies deep within you, in the land of dreams ... ... on the rock in the ocean ... ... and as you think about finding your own strength, a golden bridge forms before your eyes in this dream, leading to the rock ... ... It forms with your thought of your own strength ... ... Then you walk across the golden bridge to the rock in the ocean, which in the land of dreams can only ever be the ocean of your feelings ... ... a vast collection of feelings you once had and still carry within you

... ... also all the feelings you can have at this moment are in this ocean ... ... in the ocean of your feelings in the land of dreams ... ... You reach the rock, which stands like a stable fortress in this ocean ... ... You stand in the middle of the rock and look out over the ocean ... ... Fog rises over the ocean of feelings ... ... and in the fog, you can gradually recognize images ... ... images like on a screen ... ... They show events and memories of your life ... ... You see images from your childhood ... ... images from your youth ... ... and images from your adult life ... ... but slowly, very specific images come forward and become clearer over the water of the ocean ... ... images from a time when you had to overcome something difficult ... ... Maybe you had to overcome something as a child that was very hard for you ... ... it might have been something seemingly small but very big for you ... ... Maybe you overcame an obstacle ... ... climbed over a fence or up a tree ... ... It could also be that as a teenager, you overcame an iron boundary in sports ... ... or the boundary of your shyness ... ... or as an adult, you achieved something that was only possible with a lot of perseverance and self-overcoming ... ... You look at what you once overcame ... ... Maybe many events come to mind

… … or some very special ones … … possibly just one that was particularly important … … But whatever you overcame, you always had to overcome yourself to do so … … a form of fear that was surely different from panic, but still fear … … fear of failure … … or fear of humiliation … … or a specific fear that only you know … … You see the images over the water of the ocean of feelings … … You stand in the middle of this ocean on the rock that stands like a rock in the surf … … you are also like a rock in the surf, always facing your fears, including the panic … … You face it today as well … … But now, at this very moment, it is especially important to feel the feeling of overcoming once again … … Every overcoming is associated with effort … … but also with relief once the overcoming is achieved … … once a boundary is crossed … … especially the relief when overcoming inner boundaries … … But you have already overcome inner boundaries many times … … You had no other choice but to face them, so you did it successfully … … So you feel once again the feeling of this strength within you that has always been there … … You perceive it once again deeply within you … … let it become clear because it can help you again to overcome the difficult time … … to overcome the panic … …

today in the land of dreams and perhaps tomorrow in your waking life ... ... or just a little more each day of your life ... ... Then, filled with this strength of overcoming, you walk back across the golden bridge to the shore ... ... You trust that this strength works within you and for you and really helps you overcome the fear ... ... You lie down in the sand and watch the clouds in the sky ... ... They just keep moving, and you imagine the panic moving with them ... ... You can overcome it, and you will overcome it ... ... Fear moves away with the clouds ...

You feel the sense of freedom and relief deep within you ... ... and your mood becomes slowly happier and more relaxed ... ... Here in the land of dreams, anything is possible, including freedom from fear ... ... including redis

covering your own strength ... ... including your freedom forever ... ... Then you think about the fact that the land of dreams is deep within you ... ... It has always been there ... ... I am just telling you about it ...

Distribution, publication, and copying in any form are prohibited and subject to damages.

Overview of All Titles in the Series "Ten Hypnoses"

Volume 1: Smoking Cessation
Volume 2: Anxiety and Restlessness
Volume 3: Burnout
Volume 4: Reducing Overweight
Volume 5: Coping with the Past
Volume 6: Suicidal Thoughts and Attempts
Volume 7: Psycho-Oncology
Volume 8: Obsessions and Tics
Volume 9: Self-Confidence and Decision-Making
Volume 10: Grief Work
Volume 11: Psychosomatics
Volume 12: Chronic Pain
Volume 13: Depressive Thoughts
Volume 14: Panic Attacks
Volume 15: Domestic Violence, Victim Support
Volume 16: Post-Traumatic Stress
Volume 17: Exam Anxiety and Stage Fright
Volume 18: Anti-Violence Training, Offender Support
Volume 19: Addiction Tendencies
Volume 20: Social Phobia and Fear of Contact
Volume 21: Nail Biting
Volume 22: Self-Awareness and Self-Love
Volume 23: Teeth Grinding and Night Clenching
Volume 24: Feelings of Guilt
Volume 25: Fear in Crowds
Volume 26: Fear of Flying, Aviophobia
Volume 27: Fear in Enclosed Spaces, Claustrophobia
Volume 28: Tinnitus, Ear Noises
Volume 29: Fear of Heights
Volume 30: Neurodermatitis

Copying, publishing, and sharing with third parties are only permitted with the written consent of the author. Please observe the notes on copyright and usage.

Volume 31: Finding Inner Balance
Volume 32: Overcoming Loneliness
Volume 33: Fear of Illness, Hypochondria
Volume 34: Anticipatory Anxiety, Fear of Fear
Volume 35: Jealousy in Relationships
Volume 36: Driving Anxiety
Volume 37: New Start after Separation
Volume 38: Fear of Injections
Volume 39: Heart Anxiety Neurosis
Volume 40: Overcoming Resentment and Anger
Volume 41: Resolving Blockages and Positive Thinking
Volume 42: Stress Reduction, Stress Management
Volume 43: Body Relaxation
Volume 44: Deep Relaxation
Volume 45: Fear of the Dark
Volume 46: Falling Asleep and Staying Asleep
Volume 47: Compulsive Buying
Volume 48: Restless Legs Syndrome
Volume 49: Bulimia
Volume 50: Anorexia
Volume 51: Overcoming Nightmares
Volume 52: Imagined Deformity
Volume 53: Overcoming Distrust, Finding Trust
Volume 54: Processing Failures
Volume 55: Humiliation, Emotional Hurt
Volume 56: Distressing Compassion, Vicarious Suffering
Volume 57: Self-Forgiveness
Volume 58: Self-Awareness, Self-Confidence
Volume 59: Saying No
Volume 60: Assertiveness
Volume 61: Setting Boundaries and Self-Assertion
Volume 62: Decision-Making Ability

- Volume 63: Success Orientation
- Volume 64: Ruminating, Circular Thinking
- Volume 65: Accepting Pregnancy
- Volume 66: Birth Preparation
- Volume 67: Spiritual Opening
- Volume 68: Joy of Life and Inner Lightness
- Volume 69: Patience and Inner Peace
- Volume 70: Fibromyalgia and Rheumatism
- Volume 71: Irritable Bowel Syndrome, Crohn's Disease
- Volume 72: Fear of Nausea, Emetophobia
- Volume 73: Stuttering and Cluttering, Speech Flow Disorders
- Volume 74: Concentration and Knowledge Anchoring
- Volume 75: Vitality and Spontaneity
- Volume 76: Searching for Meaning and Finding Goals
- Volume 77: Life Crises, Life Events
- Volume 78: Workaholism, Goal Obsession
- Volume 79: Helper Syndrome, Helpless Helpers
- Volume 80: Medication Abuse
- Volume 81: Gambling Addiction
- Volume 82: Internet Addiction, Smartphone Addiction
- Volume 83: Hoarding Disorder, Compulsive Collecting
- Volume 84: Conspiracy Thoughts, Overvalued Ideas
- Volume 85: Fear of Operations and Treatments
- Volume 86: Fear of Aging
- Volume 87: Travel Anxiety
- Volume 88: Anxiety When Urinating, Paruresis
- Volume 89: Fear of Intimacy and Togetherness
- Volume 90: Fear of Blushing
- Volume 91: Coming Out in Homosexuality
- Volume 92: Charisma Training
- Volume 93: Migraines and Chronic Headaches
- Volume 94: Overcoming Allergies, Bronchial Asthma

Volume 95: Normalizing Blood Pressure
Volume 96: Compulsive Perfectionism
Volume 97: Sports Hypnosis, Motivation
Volume 98: Sports Hypnosis, Performance Enhancement
Volume 99: Determination and Focus
Volume 100: Encountering the Inner Child
Volume 101: Cravings, Binge Eating
Volume 102: Stimulating Metabolism
Volume 103: Bipolar Mood Swings
Volume 104: Borderline, Identity Crises
Volume 105: Hypomania, Euphoria, Mania
Volume 106: Restlessness, Agitation
Volume 107: Nervous Breakdown
Volume 108: Adjustment Disorders
Volume 109: Self-Alienation, Depersonalization
Volume 110: Ending Self-Pity
Volume 111: Primary Gain of Illness
Volume 112: Secondary Gain of Illness
Volume 113: Bullying, Victim Support
Volume 114: Letting Go of Envy and Jealousy
Volume 115: Fear of Spiders, Arachnophobia
Volume 116: Fear of Dogs or Cats
Volume 117: Fear of Strangers, Xenophobia
Volume 118: Excessive Worries, Generalized Anxiety
Volume 119: Strengthening Sense of Responsibility
Volume 120: Unrequited Love, Heartache
Volume 121: Work-Life Balance
Volume 122: Letting Go of Unattainable Goals
Volume 123: Allowing and Accepting Help
Volume 124: Letting Go of Adult Children
Volume 125: Tourette Syndrome
Volume 126: Life Changes and New Starts

Volume 127: Accepting Life in a Wheelchair
Volume 128: Understanding and Overcoming Homesickness
Volume 129: Understanding and Overcoming Wanderlust
Volume 130: Dizziness, Meniere's Disease
Volume 131: Overcoming Aggression
Volume 132: Cutting and Self-Harm
Volume 133: Hair Pulling, Trichotillomania
Volume 134: Postpartum Depression
Volume 135: For Relatives of Dementia Patients
Volume 136: Self-Harm, Artificial Disorders
Volume 137: Activating Self-Healing Powers
Volume 138: Preventing Depression Relapse
Volume 139: Reactive Psychoses, Follow-Up
Volume 140: Obsessive Thoughts and Impulses
Volume 141: Compulsive Checking
Volume 142: Compulsive Counting, Symmetry Obsession
Volume 143: Compulsive Washing, Cleanliness Obsession
Volume 144: Compulsive Questioning
Volume 145: Dissociative Paralysis
Volume 146: Phantom Pain
Volume 147: Overcoming Complaining
Volume 148: Hay Fever, Pollen Allergy
Volume 149: Sexual Abuse, Victim Support
Volume 150: Standing Strong Against Sexism, #metoo
Volume 151: Binge Eating
Volume 152: Overcoming Thoughts of Revenge
Volume 153: Detachment from the Aggressor, Stockholm Syndrome
Volume 154: Courage to Separate
Volume 155: Chronic Fatigue, Exhaustion
Volume 156: Fear of the Future, Existential Anxiety
Volume 157: Excessive Worry About Children
Volume 158: Fear of Failure

Volume 159: Ending Distrust and Control
Volume 160: Dejection, Dysphoria
Volume 161: Boreout, Chronic Boredom
Volume 162: Bipolar Disorders, Relapse Prevention
Volume 163: Mania, Relapse Prevention
Volume 164: Nihilism, Feelings of Worthlessness
Volume 165: Thumb Sucking
Volume 166: Being Brave
Volume 167: Being Proud
Volume 168: Overcoming Shyness
Volume 169: Being Able to Delegate Responsibility
Volume 170: Being Able to Show Emotions
Volume 171: Letting Go of Guilt, Victim Support
Volume 172: Processing Guilt, Offender Support
Volume 173: Mood Swings, Cyclothymia
Volume 174: Lack of Drive, Vital Sadness
Volume 175: Hearing Voices with Reality Reference
Volume 176: Confident Communication
Volume 177: Standing Up for Oneself
Volume 178: Taking New Paths
Volume 179: Confident Job Application
Volume 180: No Longer Being Taken Advantage Of
Volume 181: End of Submissiveness
Volume 182: Depressive Numbness
Volume 183: Mood Drops, Affective Incontinence
Volume 184: Mood Instability
Volume 185: Somatoform Disorders
Volume 186: Stomach Ulcer, Psychosomatic
Volume 187: Accepting Amputation
Volume 188: Overcoming and Letting Go of Hatred
Volume 189: Ending Accusations
Volume 190: Allowing Tears, Being Able to Cry

Volume 191: Finding and Sorting Repressed Feelings
Volume 192: Somatoform Pain
Volume 193: Living Autonomously
Volume 194: Anhedonia, Joylessness
Volume 195: Persistent Sadness
Volume 196: Obesity, Food Addiction
Volume 197: Parents of Abused Children
Volume 198: Letting Go and Letting Be
Volume 199: Childhood Sexual Abuse
Volume 200: Fear of Loss

www.ingramcontent.com/pod-product-compliance
Lightning Source LLC
Chambersburg PA
CBHW030459220526

45464CB00006B/2577